YOUR KNOWLEDGE HAS VALUE

AF144679

- We will publish your bachelor's and master's thesis, essays and papers

- Your own eBook and book - sold worldwide in all relevant shops

- Earn money with each sale

Upload your text at www.GRIN.com
and publish for free

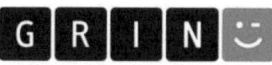

Sexual and Reproductive Health Service Utilization and Associated Factors

Among Persons with Disabilities in Addis Ababa, Ethiopia

Yonas Muluken

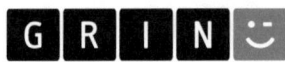

Bibliographic information published by the German National Library:

The German National Library lists this publication in the National Bibliography; detailed bibliographic data are available on the Internet at http://dnb.dnb.de.

ISBN: 9783389076712
This book is also available as an ebook.

© GRIN Publishing GmbH
Trappentreustraße 1
80339 München

Print and binding: Books on Demand GmbH, Norderstedt, Germany
Printed on acid-free paper from responsible sources.

The present work has been carefully prepared. Nevertheless, authors and publishers do not incur liability for the correctness of information, notes, links and advice as well as any printing errors.

GRIN web shop: https://www.grin.com/document/1499451

Sexual and Reproductive Health Service Utilization and Associated Factors Among Persons with Disabilities in Addis Ababa, Ethiopia

Yonas Muluken

2024

Abstract

Background: According to the world report on disability jointly issued by World Bank and WHO are estimated 17.6% of PWDs. Promoting more inclusive society and creating employment opportunities for PWDs requires improved access to basic health service needs. WHO recognize disability as a global public health issue, a human right issue and development priority. Objectives: This study is designed to investigate association factor of PWDS SRH service utilize service in health sectors in Addis Ababa in 2023. *Method*: A cross-sectional study design was used. 384 participants were selected by random sampling method in annual ceremony of FEAPD. Data were collected through structured questioner. Collected data was analyzed through Eip- info version 7. and bivariate and multivariate logistic regression analysis was employed to identify factors associated with SRH at significance is P<0.05. *Result*: PWDS perceived negative attitudes of health workers [AOR = 9.17, 95% CI: 2.81-14.09] factor for SRH service utilization. PWDS perceived poor physical accessibility and long & difficult journey to SRH service 4 [AOR, 4.11, 95% CI: 1.62-10.09] and 6[AOR, 2.83, 95%CI: 2.83 -11.30] were not utilized SRH service at significant level of P <0.01. Physical impairment were 3[AOR = 3.37, 95%CI: 1.45-9.88] risk factor of SRH utilization service than other types of disabilities.

Key words: SRH and PWDs

1. INTRODUCTION

Concerning on sexual health, there are broad challenges and problems, but female genital mutilation, sexual pleasure, violence, disease, eroticism and sexual satisfaction, sexual dysfunction, fertility and parenting, contraception are the main sexual health problem (Kira et al., 2015).

Every human being experience temporarily or permanently disability at some point in human life (Wakgari et al., 2018). According to WHO and World Bank (2011) data indicated that Peoples with Disabilities (PWDs) accounts 15-20% of the total population in developing countries. Additionally, the prevalence of disability in developing countries is higher than developed nation (WHO and World Bank, 2011). United Nations General Assembly noted that the prevalence of disabilities in developing countries estimated 80% in the year 2013 estimated 80% (Hailay et al., 2019). Similarly, children, adults and elderly PWDs in Ethiopia estimated 17.6 % (15 million) from the total population in 2011 (WHO and World Bank, 2011). Particularly, PWDs in Addis Ababa account 1.3% (36,940) from the total population of 2,739,551 in 2007 (Central Statistical Agency of Ethiopia 2013). However, both person with disabilities (PWDs) and peoples without disabilities have the similar sexual and reproductive health needs. However, PWDs often face barriers to get vital information on Sexual and Reproductive Health (SRH) service. Due to this, most PWDs unaware of their private bodies and lack of information what they do and not want to do, then they exposed for abuse (Ethiopian Center for Disability and Development, 2016).

Any human being have a right use public health service including SRH (WHO and World Bank, 2011). SRH is an vital components of the health and it is pillar for sustainable development for many countries. There are international convention right for PWDs in public health service. For instance, International Convention People for Development (ICPD) discussed the right for all men and women to utilized SRH without discrimination (WHO and World Bank, 2011). Then, United Nation Convention of articles 23 and 25 stated that PWDs have a right to utilized SRH and have the right to access to optimal reproductive and sexual health services (Ibid). Therefore, many countries implementing polices and laws of international convection, but not in line with the definition of disabilities (Unite Nation, 2013). Africa countries are facing many challenges with promoting of SRH for PWDs due to this most peoples have not awareness on components SRH service and utilized (International Conference on Population Development 1994). In many

1

developing countries, PWDs still low utilization of SRH service and related issues (WHO/UNFPA, 2009; Tigist et al., 2014). As the result, PWDs are high risk on SRH problem than person without disability (Newton-Levinson & Chandra-Mouli, 2016; Dapaah et al., 2015).

WHO/UNFPA described PWDs who have mental, long-term physical, intellectual limitation are interaction with many challenges may hinders their effective and full utilization of SRH service than persons without disabilities (WHO/UNFPA, 2009). Among over all challenges, accessibility of environments for PWDs is the main for inclusion in utilization of SRH service (World Bank and WHO, 2011). Furthermore, nature of disability, PWDs behavior, biological, institutional factors, social and environmental factors, secrete for PWDs, and the service availability and affordability were the most mentioned reasons for PWDs not utilized SRH service (Newton-Levinson & Chandra-Mouli, 2016; Dapaah et al., 2015). The most factors affecting PWDs SRH service utilization are physical inaccessible service, poverty, health facility equipment's and cost for the service, and environmental situation.

The barrier of PWDs to utilized SRH service are lack of social attention, lack of understanding, lack of support and lack of obtain basic information about SRH service (Ahumuz et al.,. 2011).. Furthermore, the negative attitudes and ignorance of unique need of PWDs, and lack of service are the main factor of PWDs for SRH service (Central Statistics Agency, 2013). Therefore, PWDs remain ignorant of basic facts about themselves to use SRH service (Ahumuz et al.,. 2011). This phenomena is similar in different area of Ethiopia. Which means PWDs are not utilized SRH like other peoples. Due to this they exposed to different problem like abortion, sexual transmitted disease. Including all these factors and other personal factors lead to poor health care seeking behavior of PWDs to reproductive health problem and PWDs has a serious consequence in later life (WHO/UNFPA, 2009; Margaret et al., 2007).

The main objective of the study is to investigate association factor of PWDS SRH service utilize service in health sectors in Addis Ababa in 2023. Thus, this study try to answer the following; question what is the level of sexual and reproductive health service utilization among persons with disabilities in Addis Ababa City Administration? And what are the main associated factor for the utilization of sexual and reproductive health service among persons with disabilities?

2. Methods and Materials

2.1 Study area

This study conducted in Addis Ababa city administration, Ethiopia. Federation of Ethiopian Associations of Persons with Disabilities (FEAPD) is well organized from district to the capital city of Addis Ababa. FEAPD have many members in Addis Ababa. Majority of members are visual impaired, hearing impaired, and physical disability.

2.2 Study design and period

Institutional based cross-sectional study was conducted using quantitative method from June 2022 to January 2023. Institution used were one Addis Ababa disabled Association. The study participants were person with disabilities of childbearing age women and men age from 15-49 years.

2.3 Study population

The source population of the study is the population of PWDs live in Addis Ababa who are member of FEAPD. The total member number of FEAPD are greater than 10,000 those who lived in Addis Ababa City Administration during the study period. The study participants were person with disabilities of childbearing age women and men age from 15-49 years.

2.4 Sample size and techniques

The study was used a probability sampling method of systematic random sampling method. FEAPD has annual meeting and celebration in August in every year. Then, FEAPD invited 635 active member participants in all Sub City in Addis Ababa. In such a way, the researcher use this big opportunity to collect the data and distribute the questionnaire for the participants at break time and at the end of the programm.

Study sample size was calculated through computer Epi Info stat calc, the sample size was determined using the formula for single population proportion. Based on a significance level of 95 % ($\alpha = 0.05$), a five percent margin of error, and an assumption of 50 % prevalence of SRH-related problems among study subjects. To estimate population proportion (P) with narrow confidence interval and high precision and when there is no prior information about the population proportion. We can determine the sample size by using the formula and p=q=0.5, p-value is 0.05.

According the formula, total sample size for the study was 384 but 10% would be added for the expected non-response, making the final sample size 422. The study was used a probability

3

sampling of systematic random sampling method. The the study response rate was 94% (398) and use for data analysis.

2.5 Data Collection instrument

The main data collection instrument was questionnaire. Alongside, socio-demographic characteristics was included in the questionnaire. The main components of the questionnaires are sexual behavior items, awareness of respondent's towards SRH service items, environmental factor items and institutional factors items and constructed for the participants.

2.6 Data collectors and collection procedures

5 data collectors (2 have sign language diploma certificate and 3 degree holders) were selected for the data collection in FEAPD ceremony festival. After selection 1 hour training were given for all data collectors by the principal investigator prior to 2 days before data collection period about the objectives of the study and how to collect the data. The overall activities were controlled by the principal investigator. Particularly, 2 data collectors were assign for hearing impaired who are did not read and write at all as well as 3 of the rest were assign for visual impaired. However, 3 program coordinators help to collect the data from PWDs at the end of the period.

2.7 Data Processing Analysis

In this study, data analysis method was employed to answering the research question. The quantitative data was analyzed by using EPI info 7 Version. The major descriptive statistics techniques was used for the questionnaire such as frequency, percentage, graph, bivariate logistic regression. The level of significant was declared at p value <0.05 and Odds ratio and 95% confidence interval used to check significant association between dependent & independent variables.

3. Result of the study

3.1 Socio-demographic characteristics of the participants

Out of 398 respondents, 186 (46.73%) were male and 212 (53.27%) were females. The respondents age 20-30 were the highest number of the respondent the median age of respondents were between 30- 40 age group. 35(8.79%) were hearing impaired, 225 (56.53%) were physical impaired, 122 (30.65%) were vision impaired, 16 (4.02%) were have other impairment.

4

Most of participants education level were elementary and secondary school 29.65% and 42.71% respectively. This means those participants did not upgrade their educational level in different factors. While, a few had 38(9.55%) of certificate and 12(3.02%) diploma and above. From occupation status, unemployment and private employments were the highest respondents (108, 27.14%) and (111, 27.89%) respectively. Among time of disability most of the respondents were early time disability (208, 52.26%). From occupation status, unemployment and private employments were the highest respondents (108, 27.14%) and (111, 27.89%) respectively.

3.2 Components of SRH services utilized by respondents

Respondents were used SRH service components but the study result indicated that most respondents had not experience to utilize SRH components.

Figure 1 shows that 335 (84%) were not used SRH service components. While very a few respondents were used SRH component service. For instance family planning, voluntary counselling and testing for HIV/AIDS and Sexual Transmitted Infections (STIs) treatment and diagnosis were used by respondents 21(5%), 12 (3%) and 13(3%) respectively. Almost none respondents were not used Other SRH component services compare to the respondent numbers however respondents were used 3(1%) from those SRH component services.

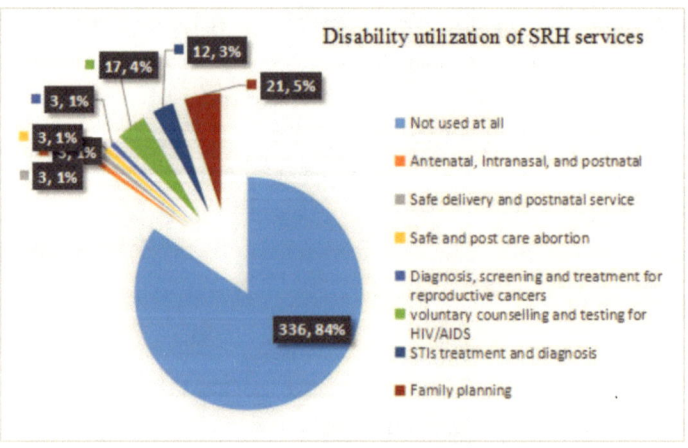

Source: *survey data 2024*

Figure 1 Components of SRH services utilized by respondents

5

3.3 Respondents understanding of SRH service place

According to the assessment of the study on where SRH service were given that perceived by the respondents were shows that most respondents had understanding about where SRH service place (69 male and 52 female) which is available in hospital, government health center, pharmacy, private clinic and NGO service.

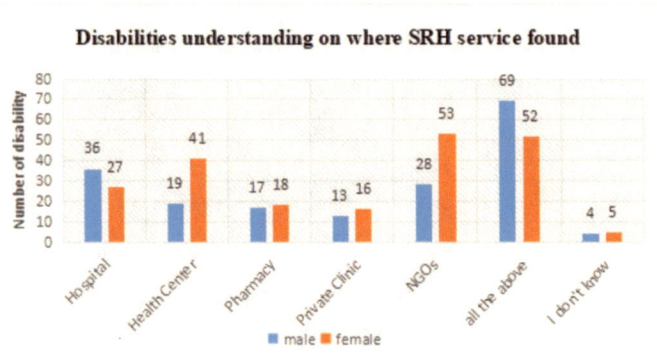

Source: *survey data 2024*

Figure 2 Respondents perception on SRH service places

The above figure illustrated that 36 male and 27 female were perceived SRH service found in hospital. Beside of this 19 male and 41 females were also had understanding of where SRH service given. While a few 4 male and 5 female were did not know where SRH service given. Generally the above figure shows that most respondents had knowledge where SRH service given.

3.4 Respondents SRH service place perception and SRH utilization

Regarding on the above finding, the study results show that respondents experience to utilize SRH service illustrated in figure 3.

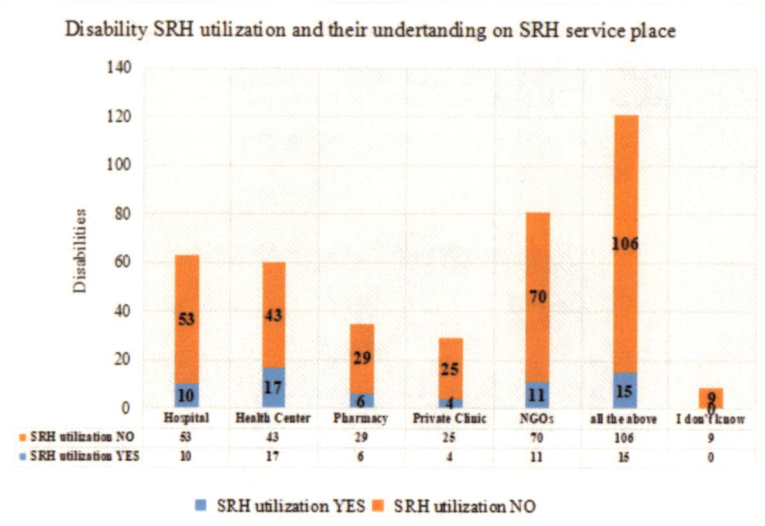

Source: survey data 2024

Figure 3 Respondents perception on SRH service places and utilization of SRH service

Figure 3 shows that respondents know and understand where SRH service is given and their experience of use SRH service was bad. It means most respondents had awareness of SRH service place but they did not utilize the service. The data indicated that 15 respondents were use SRH service among 121 respondents that had well know SRH service is given all health organizations. Contrary, respondents had not knowledge about where SRH service given they were not used SRH service. Most respondents were not use SRH while a few 63 (15.8%) were use SRH service among the respondents. But 97.7% of respondents know where SRH service is given.

3.5 Factors associated with utilization of SRH services among PWDS

The study attempted to correlate socio-demographic factors and awareness about SRH service, environmental factor, institutional factor and sexual behavior of PWDS with reproductive health service utilization among PWDS in Addis Ababa. Those correlation were employed by bivariate and multivariate logistic regression.

3.5.1 Factors associated with SRH service utilization among PWDS socio-demographic

Table 1 PWDS socio-demographic factor on SRH service utilization in Addis Ababa

Socio-demographic characteristic		SRH Utilization		AOR (95%CI)	COR (95%CI)	P Value
		No %	Yes %			
Gender	Male	181(54.19)	5(7.81)	1.701(.99-2.92)	0.558(.342-1.01)	0.54
	Female	153(45.81)	59(92.19)	1		
Age	15-20	42(12.57)	6(9.38)	2.81(1.11- 7.12)	0.58(0.37- 0.89)	0.03
	20-30	155(46.41)	11(17.19)	5.66(2.77 - 11.5)	0.95(0.63– 1.41)	0.00
	30-40	102(30.54)	41(64.06)	1		
	40-50	35(10.48)	6(9.38)	2.34(0.92 -5.99)	0.56(0.36 -0.86)	0.10
Types disability	Hearing impairment	30(8.98)	5(7.81)	3.60(0.9 - 14.39)	0.69(0.34-1.43)	0.07
	Physical impairment	191(57.19)	34(53.13)	3.37(1.15-9.88)	0.96 (0.63-1.48)	0.03
	Vision impairment	103(30.84)	19(29.69)	3.25(0.92-9.99)	0.86(0.52-1.44)	0.04
	Other impairment	10(2.99)	6(9.38)	1		
Time of disability	From birth	33(9.88)	9(14.06)	1		
	Early childhood	173(51.80)	35(54.69)	1.35(0.59-3.07)	0.89(0.59 - 1.37)	0.5
	In later life	128(38.32)	20(31.25)	1.75(0.73-4.19)	1.08(0.75-1.45)	0.32
Education level	Cannot read write	48(14.37)	12(18.75)	0.36(0.04-3.09)	0.87(0.45-1.68)	0.68
	Elementary	101(30.24)	17(26.56)	0.54(0.07-4.46)	1.19(0.68-2.095)	1.00
	Secondary	143(42.81)	27(42.19)	0.48(0.06-3.89)	1.05(0.65-1.70)	0.691
	Certificate	31(79.28)	7(10.94)	0.40(0.04-3.65)	1.00(0.45-2.24)	0.66
	Diploma and above	11(3.29)	1(1.56)	1		

** Statistically significant at P<0.01 and * statistically significant at P<0.05

Table 1 results shows that physical impairment and visual impairment were not likely to utilize SRH service than other types of disability. Physical impairment were 3[AOR = 3.37, 95%CI: 1.45-9.88] risk factor of SRH utilization service than other types of disabilities. Similarly, visual impairment were also 3 times factor association of did not utilize SRH service (AOR, 3.25, 95%CI: 0.92-9.99). Contrary, hearing impairment and other types of impairment were not association factor if SRH service.

The other factor association of SRH service were age of PWDS. 20-30 age of PWDS were the higher association factor of utilization of SRH service, which were 6 times likely did not use SRH service than other age categories [AOR = 5.66. 95% CI: 2.77- 11.54]. Beside of this, the age categories 15 -20 of PWDS were a risk factor of SRH service utilization (AOR, 2.81, 95% CI: 1.11- 7.12). While, other age categories of PWDS were not association factor of SRH service.

3.5.2 Factors associated with SRH service utilization among PWDS respondents, in Addis Ababa

Table 2 Disabilities Sexual behavior association factor with SRH service utilization

Sexual behavior Factor		SRH Utilization		AOR (95%CI)	COR (95%CI)	P Valu
		No %	Yes %			
Have sexual Partner	Yes	245(73.4)	62(96.9)	3.56(1.49-8.55)	1.65(0.18-15.2)	1.00
	NO	2(3.1)	89(26.7)	1	1	
Sexual intercourse with your sexual partner in 12 month	Yes	239(71.6)	56(87.5)	1.23(0.14-12.15)	2.78(1.27-6.05)	1.00
	No	95(24.4)	8(12.5)	1	1	
Use condom in 12 month	Yes	176(52.7)	44(68.8)	0.36(0.04-3.29)	0.51(0.29-0.89)	0.64
	No	158(47.3)	20(31.3)	1	1	
Used contraceptive in 12 month	Yes	62(18.6)	18(28.1)	1	1	1.00
	No	272(81.4)	46(71.9)	1.06(0.17-6.49)	0.87(0.50-1.52)	

** Statistically significant at P<0.001 and * statistically significant at P<0.05

The above table results indicates that sexual behavior of the PWDS which is contraceptive user, sexual partners, condom user and sexual intercourse of disabilities were not associated factor of SRH service utilization. While, both PWDS had sexual partner and use condom were association with SRH service utilization among other sexual behavior of disabilities.

Table 3 Environment factors on SRH utilization association factor with SRH service utilization

Environment factors on SRH utilization		SRH Utilization		AOR (95%CI)	COR (95%CI)	P Valu
		No %	Yes %			
Poor physical accessibility (Ramps, bath rooms, examination bed and elevators)	Yes	306(91.6)	6(9.4)	4.11(1.62-10.09)	1.9(0.91-3.7)	0.00
	No	28(8.4)	58(90.6)	1	1	
Long and difficult journey to SRH service	Yes	304(91.0)	9(14.0)	6.33(2.83- 11.3)	4.72(2.3-8.4)	0.00
	No	30(8.9)	55(85.9)	1	1	
Long queues	Yes	59(17.7)	9(14.0)	1.61(0.17-14.77)	1.38(0.72-2.66)	1.00
	No	275(82.3)	55(85.9)	1	1	

** Statistically significant at P<0.001 and * statistically significant at P<0.05

Table 3 result indicated that PWDS perceived poor physical accessibility and long & difficult journey to SRH service 4 [AOR, 4.11, 95% CI: 1.62-10.09] and 6[AOR, 2.83, 95%CI: 2.83 - 11.30] were not utilized SRH service at significant level of P <0.01 than who did not perceived those. However, long and difficult journey to utilize SRH service were the highest risk factor of disabilities. Contrary, long queues were not the factor that PWDS used SRH service.

9

Table 4 Institutional factors association with SRH utilization of PWDS

Institutional factor on SRH utilization		SRH Utilization		AOR (95%CI)	COR (95%CI)	P Value
		No %	Yes %			
High cost for SRH service	Yes	267(79.9)	31(48.4)	2.81(0.46-6.00)	1.60(0.25-3.60)	0.00
	No	67(20.0)	33(51.6)	1	1	
Negative attitudes of health workers	Yes	265(79.3)	26(40.6)	9.17(2.81-14.09)	7.41(4.16-13.19)	0.00
	No	69(20.6)	38(59.4)	1	1	
Lack of confidentiality by the expertise	Yes	301(90.1)	24(37.5)	5.33(3.83-9.30)	2.84(0.92-5.86)	0.00
	No	33(9.9)	40(62.5)	1	1	
Poor of accessible information communication methods	Yes	314(94.0)	3(4.7)	6.33(5.83-8.30)	3.01(1.91-8.35)	0.00
	No	20(5.0)	61(95.3)	1	1	
Poor experience of health workers to handle PWDS	Yes	226(67.7)	41(64.1)	1	1	0.41
	No	108(32.3)	23(35.9)	0.49(0.05-4.49)	1.17(0.67-2.05)	

* Statistically significant at P<0.001 and * statistically significant at P<0.05

PWDS perceived Poor communication were 6[AOR= 6.33, 95% CI: 5.83-8.30] times more likely did not use SRH service than those who were not perceived at the significant level p<0.05. The major and the second association factor were disabilities lack confidentiality by the SRH expertise thus PWDS perceived lack confidentiality by the SRH expertise 5 times more likely did not utilize SRH service than who were not perceived lack confidentiality [AOR, 5.33, 95%CI: 3.83 - 9.30].

PWDS perceived negative attitudes of health workers and high cost for SRH service were not use SRH service than who did not perceived those [AOR = 9.17, 95% CI: 2.81-14.09] and [AOR = 2.81, 95% CI: 0.46 - 6.00] respectively. While, Poor experience of health workers to handle PWDS perceived by disabilities were not associated factor with not used SRH service.

Ironically, Poor of accessible information communication methods, lack of confidentiality by the expertise, poor physical accessibility and long and difficult journey to SRH service perceived by PWDS were higher score that factor on not utilize SRH service than who were not perceived those. Beside of this the second factor associated with SRH service were negative attitudes of health workers, high cost for SRH service that perceived by PWDS than who were not perceived those. Nevertheless, disabilities perceived poor experience of health workers to handle PWDS and long queues were not factor for SRH service utilization. In addition, sexual intercourse, use

10

of contraceptive behavior, sexual partner, use condom and PWDS awareness on SRH service were not associated factor for SRH service utilization.

Table 5 PWDS awareness on SRH service association factor with SRH service utilization

Awareness factors on SRH utilization		SRH Utilization		AOR (95%CI)	COR (95%CI)	P Valu
		No %	Yes %			
Sexual health education and prevention information for young people, single adults, and couples	Yes	66(19.8)	15(23.4)	0.45(0.07-2.80)	0.80(0.43-1.52)	0.73
	No	268(80.24)	49(76.6)	1	1	
Sexuality counseling for the client's sexual health concerns or needs, and desired sexuality, reproductive or contraceptive preferences	Yes	199(59.6)	40(62.5)	1.03(0.11-9.47)	0.7(10.37-1.33)	1.00
	No	135(40.4)	24(37.5)	1	1	
Voluntary counseling, testing, treatment and follow-up for STIs, including HIV	Yes	314(94.1)	60(93.8)	0.23(0.02-2.29)	0.75(0.27-2.08)	0.26
	No	20(5.99)	4(6.25)	1	1	
Identification and referral for victims of sexual and other forms of violence	Yes	43(12.87)	5(7.81)	0.76(0.08-7.07)	1.42(0.58-3.51)	1.00
	No	291(87.1)	59(92.2)	1	1	
Diagnosis, screening, treatment and follow-up for reproductive cancers, and associated infertility	Yes	130(38.9)	26(49.6)	0.99(0.11-9.16)	0.88(0.44-1.71)	1.00
	No	204(61.1)	38(59.4)	1	1	
Antenatal, intra- natal and post-natal care for the pregnant women	Yes	275(82.6)	55(85.9)	0.35(0.06-2.15)	1.01(0.49-2.05)	0.24
	No	58(17.4)	9(14.0)	1	1	
Safe abortion to the full extent of the law	Yes	72(21.6)	12(18.8)	1.17(0.13-10.77)	1.19(0.60-2.35)	1.00
	No	262(78.4)	52(81.3)	1	1	
Post-abortion care, including provision of contraceptive information, counseling and methods	Yes	126(37.7)	24(37.5)	0.90(0.77-1.07)	0.04(0.02-0.08)	0.12
	No	208(62.3)	40(62.5)	1	1	

** Statistically significant at P<0.001 and * statistically significant at P<0.05

The above table result shows that PWDs awareness on SRH service were high. While, PWDs awareness on SRH service were insignificant associated factor of SRH service utilization.

To sum up, according to the study result illustrated that environment factor were the major associated factor PWDs to utilize SRH service than other factors. On the other hand, institutional factors were the second major associated factor PWDs to utilize SRH service.

11

4. Conclusion and Recommendation

The study showed sexual and reproductive health service utilization of PWD were found to be very low. According to the finding of this study the service accessibility, poor physical environment, information communication barrier could be main reasons for not utilized the SRH service among person with disabilities. While, negative attitude of the health care provides, long and difficult journey to get SRH, gender, types of disability and some age group status was significantly associated factor of PWDs SRH service utilization. Other variables like awareness on SRH service and service delivery point and sexual behavior were not association factor of PWDs SRH service utilization. Therefore, it needs a great effort and attention of all the concerned body to increase the SRH service utilization among PWDs by designing and implementing appropriate SRH service for PWD. Additionally, the nationwide research also needed to gain more accurate data on total population of PWDs to develop and implement effective, inclusive and effective strategies to improve the current SRH situation of PWDs. Based on the result of this study, the study forwarded the following recommendations:

✧ Minster of Health better to develop information communication related material for all kind of disabilities to easily communicate and understanding the program.
✧ Minster of Health and NGO's better to focus on making SRH service and giving the facilities more disability friendly.
✧ Policy makers better try to incorporate at all level PWDs right of SRH and mainstreaming the PWDs issue.
✧ Minster of Health and NGO's health organization should work collaboratively to developed PWDs inclusive in all SRH program.

Limitation of this study

- Since this study examines personal and sensitive issues, obtaining honest responses among person with disabilities it have been difficult. Therefore this data might have prone to respondent bias.
- The SRH service utilization was assessed without considering specific disability type may be have implication in the use of SRH service so that if study conducted on specific disabilities have different finding.

- Other barriers on sexual and reproductive health service utilization from provider's side were not assessed in this study.
- The quantitative study design did not allow for probing or searching into certain areas which, means the findings may not be generalization to the overall Ethiopian person with disabilities. So I strongly recommend qualitative study or mixed type for this kind of sensitive and personal issues.

Reference

Ahumuz et al.,. (2011). *Challenges in accessing sexual and reproductive health services by people with physical disabilities in Kampala,* Uganda. Reproductive health 2014 11:59.

Anna Newton-Levinson JSL, and Venkatraman Chandra-Mouli. (2016). Sexually Transmitted Infection Services for Adolescents and Youth in Low- and Middle-Income Countries Perceived and Experienced Barriers to Accessing Care. *Journal of Adolescent Health; 59 7 e16* http://creativecommons.org/licenses/by-nc-nd/4.0/.

Central Statistics Agency. (2013). *Representation of Persons with Disabilities: A Review of National Surveys on Disability Statistics*

Ethiopian Center for Disability and Development (ECDD) and DKT Ethiopia (2016). *Assessment of sexual and reproductive health products & services use by persons with disabilities.*

Hailay Gebreyesus, Mebrahtu Teweldemedhin and Abebe Mamo. (2019). *Determinants of reproductive health Services utilization among rural female Adolescents in Asgede-Tsimbla district Northern Ethiopia* . Article Google Scholar.

Jonathan Mensah Dapaah, Seth Christopher Yaw Appiah, Eric Badu, Bernard Obeng,Victoria Ampiah. (2015). *Does Facility Based Sexual and Reproductive Health Services Meet the Needs of Young Persons? Views from Cross Section of Ghanaian Youth.* Advances in Sexual Medicine.

Kira L., Alexander D.,Jesusa Ma., Marco J., Zayas L., Gill A. (2015). *Sexual and reproductive Health Service for women with disability.* BMC women's Health, 15; 87.

Margaret A. Nosekand Darrell K. Simmons Baylor. (2007). People with Disabilities as a Health Disparities Population: The Case of Sexual and Reproductive Health Disparities. *Californian Journal of Health Promotion.*

Maxwell J., Belser JW.and David DA. (2007). *Health Hand Book for women with disability.* Berkely, CA Hesperian Foundation.

Tigist Alemu Kassa, Tobias Luck, Samuel Kinde Birru, and Steffi G. Riedel-Heller. (2014). *Sexuality and Sexual Reproductive Health of Disabled Young People in Ethiopia.* PubMed.

Unite Nation. (2013). *Convention on the right of person with disabilities.* http//www.UN.org./disabilities/convention/conventionfull.shtml.

Wakgari Binu1, Taklu Marama, Mulusew Gerbaba and Melese Sinaga. (2018) *Sexual and reproductive health services utilization and associated factors among secondary school students in Nekemte Towm, Ethiopia.* Article Google Scholar

WHO/UNFPA. (2009). *Promoting Sexual and Reproductive health for persons with disabilities.* WHO /UNFPA Guidance not.

World Bank and World Health Organization. (2011). *World Report on Disability*, Washington, D. C.